Healthy Eating

Introduction to Vegetables

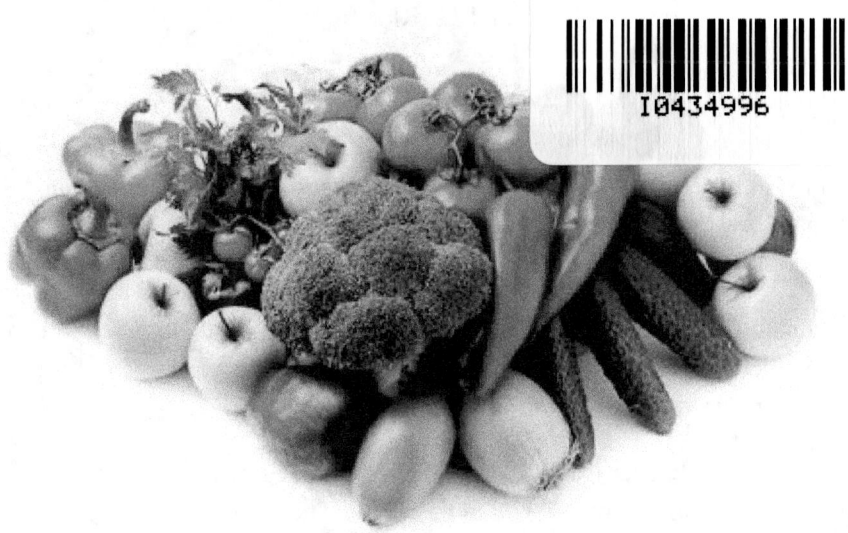

Natural Health Series

Dueep J. Singh

Mendon Cottage Books

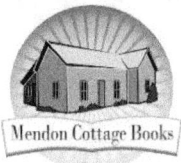

JD-Biz Publishing

Disclaimer

The information is this book is provided for informational purposes only. It is not intended to be used and medical advice or a substitute for proper medical treatment by a qualified health care provider. The information is believed to be accurate as presented based on research by the author.

The contents have not been evaluated by the U.S. Food and Drug Administration or any other Government or Health Organization and the contents in this book are not to be used to treat cure or prevent disease.

The author or publisher is not responsible for the use or safety of any diet, procedure or treatment mentioned in this book. The author or publisher is not responsible for errors or omissions that may exist.

Warning

The Book is for informational purposes only and before taking on any diet, treatment or medical procedure, it is recommended to consult with your primary health care provider.

Check out some of the other Healthy Gardening Series books at Amazon.com

Gardening Series on Amazon

Check out some of the other Health Learning Series books at Amazon.com

Health Learning Series on Amazon

Table of Contents

INTRODUCTION TO VEGETABLES — 1

INTRODUCTION — 4

VEGETABLE CUISINE IN ASIA — 8

INDIGENOUS VEGETABLES — 10

CABBAGES AND POTATOES — 12

POTATO ROSTI — 13

VEGETABLE-BASED DISHES IN EUROPE — 14

WHY COOK VEGETABLES IN SLICES — 16

LEAF WRAPPED FOODS — 17

TRADITIONAL CABBAGE ROLLS — 19

SAUERKRAUT — 20

KIMCHI-OR FERMENTED RADISH/CABBAGE — 22

ARTICHOKES — 24

CHOOSING AND EATING ARTICHOKES — 25

WHITE SAUCE FOR ARTICHOKES — 26

PEAS — 27

TRADITIONAL PEAS PUDDING — 28

DOLMA — 29

SAUTÉ FENNEL — 31

CONCLUSION — 32

AUTHOR BIO — 33

PUBLISHER — 43

Introduction

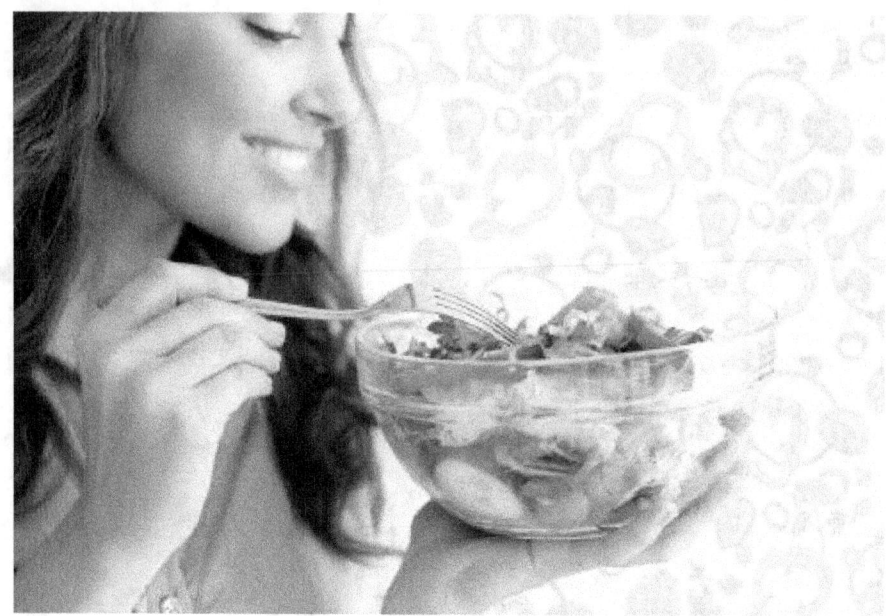

Someone once asked me whether I was a vegetarian, and when I said that I had tried vegetarianism for about five years, she asked me whether I found some improvement in my health. And even my mental and spiritual behavior and outlook?

As she is a strict vegetarian, and is rather fanatical about promoting vegetarianism in her circle. She was a bit disappointed when I said, well, I can take it or leave it, and I did not find any great change in health, when I was a vegetarian, and then one fine day I decided to go back to my state of omnivorous grazing, which included everything from vegetables, roots, bark, leaves to snakes and snails and oxtails.

Well, let me admit that I was taking a Mickey out of her. Vegetarianism had improved my health considerably, as well as made me feel more youthful, energetic, and had even improved the texture of my skin and hair. But I was not going to admit that to her. And then I had digressed back to animal tissue, and found that the extra toxic waste build up in my body had brought my health level back to what it was previously before I had started on a fully vegetarian diet.

Also, I did not want to admit to her another rather tricky matter of personal hygiene. When I was on a vegetarian diet, eating just vegetables, so, all right, I used to sweat as much as any other average person living in a moist, hot and muggy, humid atmosphere in the summer. But the sweat did not give out a displeasing odor at all. In fact, it was almost like the body was getting rid of extra water through the skin.

So for all those people, who are so used to using lots of deodorants, in the summer, in order to get rid of that pong, try eating a fruit and vegetable diet in summer, without any vestige of meat or spices. You will be surprised at the nearly immediate and visible and very clearly apparent change, within two – three days.

As for my tendency of losing my temper at the drop of a hat, believe it or not, in the five years when I practiced being a vegetarian on a total fruit and vegetable and cereals diet, I was a much calmer person, and whether that is due to autosuggestion or just because I was growing up more tolerant is a thing of which I am not quite certain!

I am definitely not advocating vegetarianism, if you are not inclined to change your eating habits. However, I intend to introduce more vegetables as a welcome addition to your diet.

Depending on the place in which you live, there is a wide-ranging variety and choice of fresh vegetables which are going to be available to you all year round, unless you are living in the frozen reaches of the South Pole and the North Pole. Even there, you are going to get frozen vegetables.

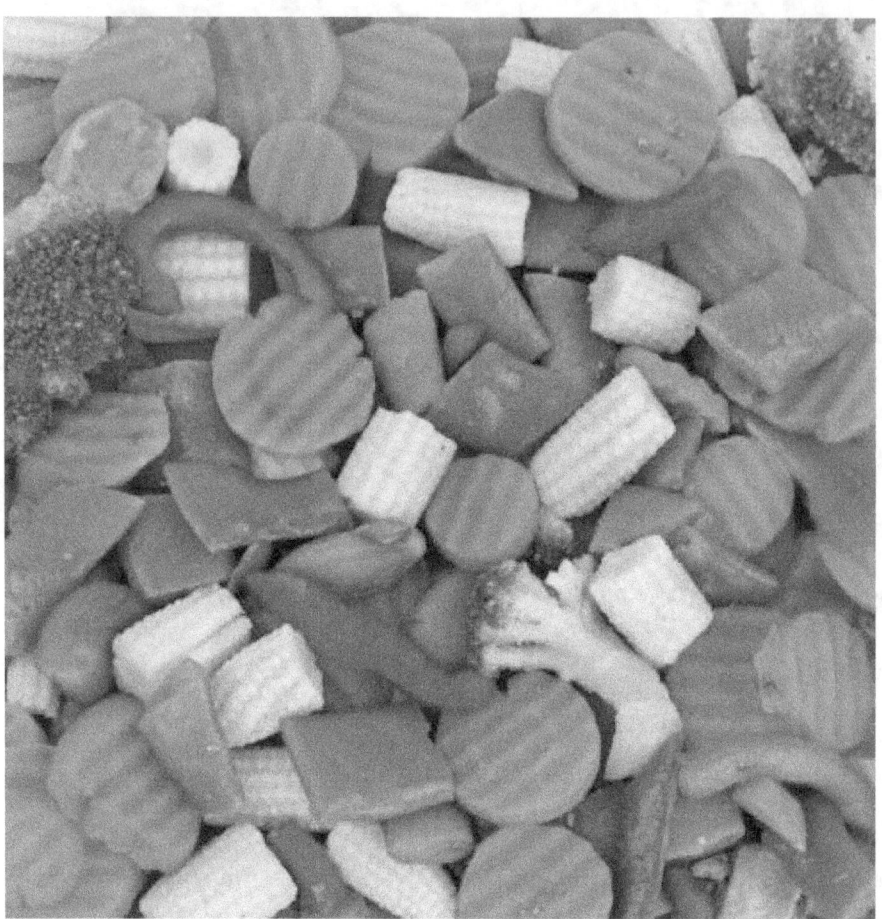

Frozen vegetables are available all over the world, but fresh vegetables are always the better and healthier option.

I remember some Air Force pilot acquaintances, who were posted up high in the mountains. Anybody going for a month's leave, back home, and in the claims, down there, was immediately given a long list from all of his friends and it would be blood for breakfast if he did not come back with every item in the list brought back safely. These items included homemade food.

This list also included vegetables like greens, yellows, oranges, reds and any other color in between. Any sort of vegetable would do, because it was the change in fare, from the monotonous and ubiquitous potato.

This was 20 years ago, and greenhouses in the mountains, allow these hardy pilots to gain access to fresh vegetables throughout the year. But this should show you that things that we consider usual, and normal, and part of our daily fair, or considered to be exotic and as precious as the spices of yore in some parts of the world.

Greengrocers, and supermarkets are importing more and more vegetables which ones were considered to be exotic. For that we can give thanks to the fast transport system, which allows me to eat asparagus, kale, artichokes, broccoli, and Brussels Sprouts in areas where once upon a time there were just photographs in a book, and one wondered how they tasted.

Thanks to easy access to these vegetables, our diets have become more and more varied. That means that once, when we stuck to our own traditional diet, because that meant that we were using the vegetables easily available to us in our local market, now we can try experimenting with global cuisine.

So that means I can try Chinese water chestnuts in a recipe or Bok Choy. I can also try lemongrass, and recipes using indigenous Thai vegetables like kangkong, water mimosa, spiny gourd or hairy eggplant. So, thanks to the easy access to a number of vegetables, which were once indigenous, I can cultivated a global palate.

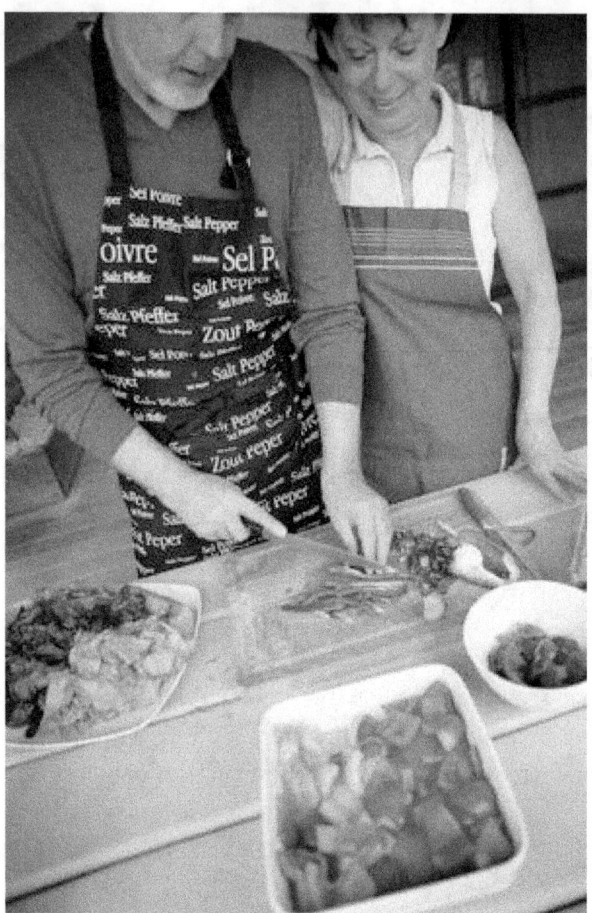

Vegetable Cuisine in Asia

China is one country, which has a wealth of indigenous vegetables, and bamboo shoots and ginger are some of the global contributions, to which we should be grateful to this land.

This country, like a number of other countries of the East has enormous vegetable resources, and even though little meat is used, – for millenniums, the cuisine of many Eastern countries has been predominantly vegetarian, depending on herbs, spices, vegetable and fruit as well as cereals to make up their daily fare of the people living there – the absence of meat is not noticed because the flavor and freshness of the vegetables are preserved so beautifully.

However, in traditional Chinese cuisine, the usage of milky, buttery and creamy sauces are not often favored, as they are favored in Western cuisine.

Vegetables are often cooked in pans, in oil. Water is used very rarely accept for a supplement to oils and sauces like soy. Along with the bamboo shoots and bean shoots, which are used in this cuisine very often, the Chinese also use soya beans, Tiger Lily cups, even the gelatinous lining of nests, tree – fungi, and of course many cereals, including rice, millet and noodle mixtures.

Meat, chicken and fish are diced very carefully, in tiny pieces, slivers and scraps. These are cooked only just sufficiently and with every effort to retain each and every ingredient's aroma and flavor. These are then steam cooked and braised in stock, so that the flavor can be retained with these gentle cooking methods. Fast boiling is definitely not accepted, nor is it used very often in traditional Chinese cookery.

In the Indian subcontinent, there are many vegetables, which come in the exotic category, when seen through Western eyes. These include Lotus roots, okra, bitter gourd, white pumpkin, drumstick beans, bananas, neem flowers, fenugreek [which is normally used as an Herb in the West, but is used as a vegetable in the subcontinent, like spinach] and yam.

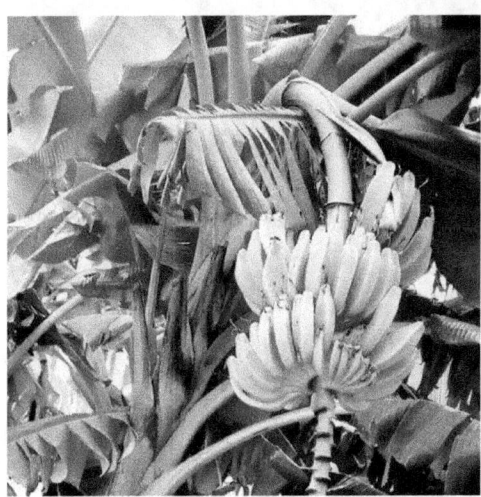

Bananas, even though considered by most people to be a fruit are part of traditional cuisine, cooked as vegetables in many parts of the world.

Indigenous Vegetables

There are a number of factors which influence the outcome of shortages and abundances of vegetables in a particular area. These factors are going to include climatic conditions, and also agricultural conditions.

For example, you are not going to find mushrooms very often in Spain. If you are in South Africa, you are going to get an overabundance of mealies which are also known under the name of sweet corn or maize. This is a part of the staple diet, and is used in different preparations. It is either boiled with butter and salt. Sometimes you pulp it and blend it with eggs, butter, seasonings, and seasonings, and then bake it.

So when you are used to eating potatoes, in copious quantities in other parts of the world, in South Africa, you are going to be eating mealies. On the other hand, you are not going to get fresh sweet corn very often in England and many other cold European countries, where it is still considered to be a luxury item.

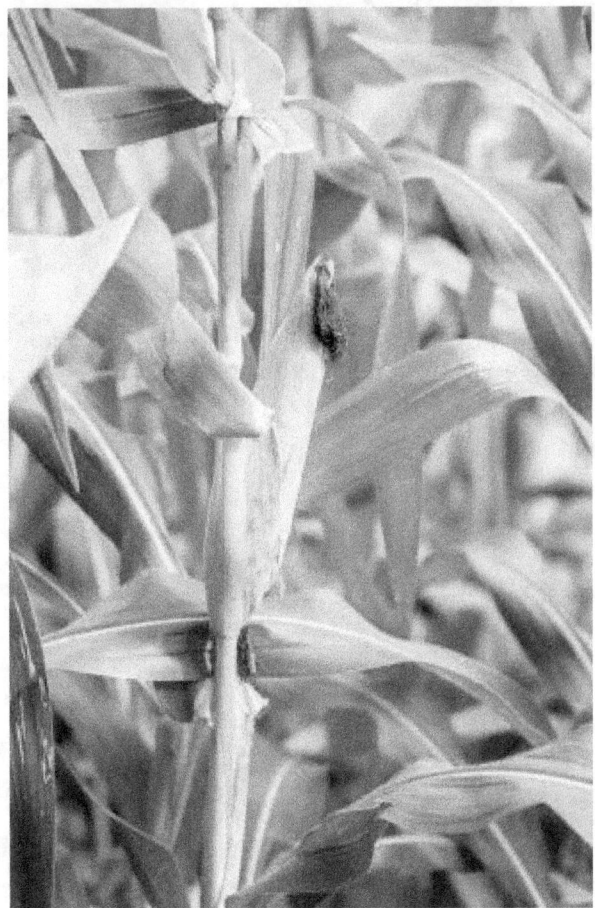

Mealies, such an important part of man's staple diet for millenniums, especially in Africa and in other parts of the world, is just another name for ordinary corn or maize.

Cabbages and Potatoes

Once upon a time cabbages and potatoes were considered to be the staple diet of people living in areas, where there was a history of poverty or the land suffered from war or deprivation very often. So even though these two vegetables are considered to be a staple poor man's diet, you cannot forget that even in times of plenty, they are used extensively to fill hungry stomachs.

In fact, the Irish were so used to the potato, that a couple of centuries ago, when a complete potato crop was wiped out due to disease, millions starved. That is because they had not thought of planting anything else which could be a vegetable standby.

Potato Rosti

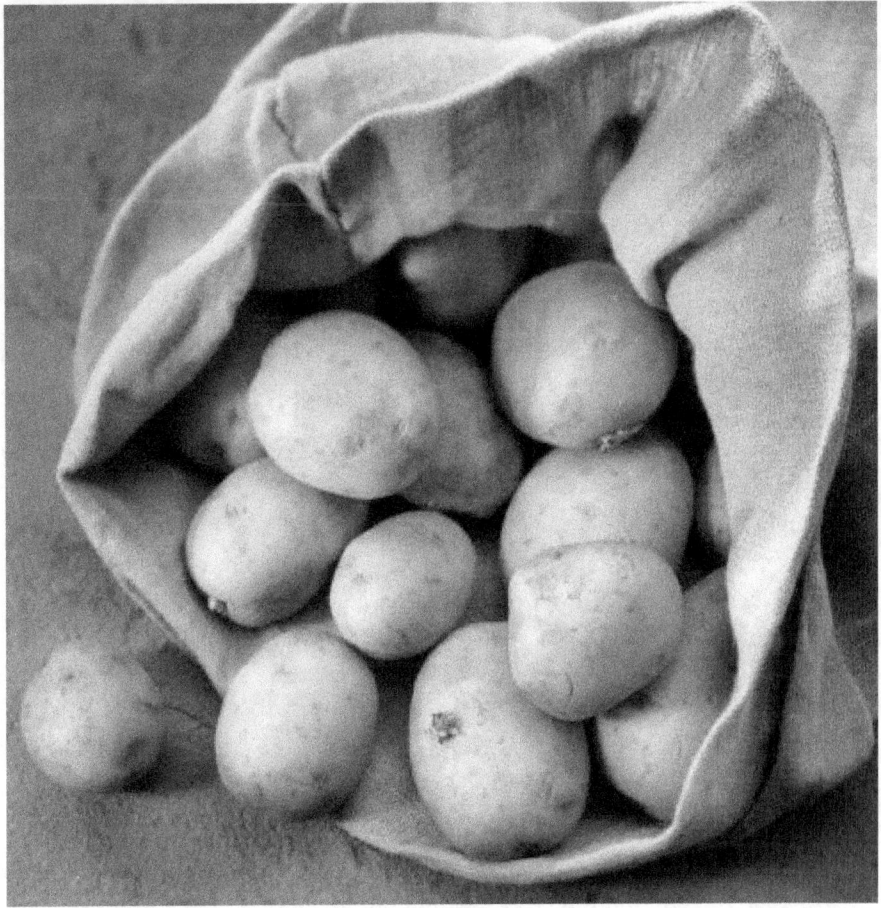

This is a popular traditional dish in Switzerland when the potatoes are panfried.

To make this, you need 2 ½ cups of grated and raw potatoes, one onion, grated, two eggs, 1 teaspoon full of salt, a pinch of pepper, pinch of nutmeg, and 2 tablespoons full of cooking fat.

Combine the grated raw potatoes, onions, eggs, salt, pepper and nutmeg. Melt 1 tablespoon of the fat in bottom of heated frying pan. Pour in the potato mixture. Cook slowly until the underside is well browned.

With a knife or narrow spatula, loosen the sides and bottom, then invert a plate or fat lid over the pan. Lift the half cooked potatoes out on the plate.

Add another tablespoonful of fat to the pan and slide the potatoes back in the pan to brown the other side.

This is going to take 15 – 20 minutes of cooking time. Cut into quarters to serve 4 people.

Vegetable-based dishes in Europe

Austria, Germany and Switzerland, and all the adjoining countries of Europe are the homes of many traditional cabbage recipes, but the dishes with cabbage as a main ingredient are generally gaining importance over plain boiled cabbage all over the world. So think sauerkraut recipes, in which white and red cabbage is going to be served with herbs and seasoning. There is also cabbage with apples, and stuffed cabbages – recipes originating in France.

In Scandinavia, most of the vegetables that are known are served in a creamy and savory sauces, which make up Scandinavian cuisine. The Scandinavians love Apple and cabbage combinations, chestnuts used as vegetables, creamed mushrooms, various forms of onions and brown potatoes, cauliflowers with egg and cheese sauces, and nourishing potato dumplings.

In Finland, even now, fresh and green vegetables are still something of a luxury, but you can get plenty of tinned and frozen vegetables very easily. Greenhouses are being made to provide these fresh green vegetables to the general public, but even so, the struggle is slow and steady against the harsh and bitter climate of that particular area. Nevertheless, their cuisine is also very innovative, with plenty of creative combinations like egg and onion combinations or egg and cabbage puddings.

Also, the ladies of Finland are adept in making lots of pickles, including beetroot pickles. So unless one is really very finicky and choosy, and is adamant about eating fresh vegetables, one does not really find any sort of "vegetable deprivation" while eating out here on local fare.

In Ireland, "colcannon" is a typical combination of potatoes and cabbage. The potato is made into a creamy purée, and the cabbages precooked. To this is added spring onions and chopped bacon, if you want it or it is available. The mixture is then fried as a pancake and browned on both sides.

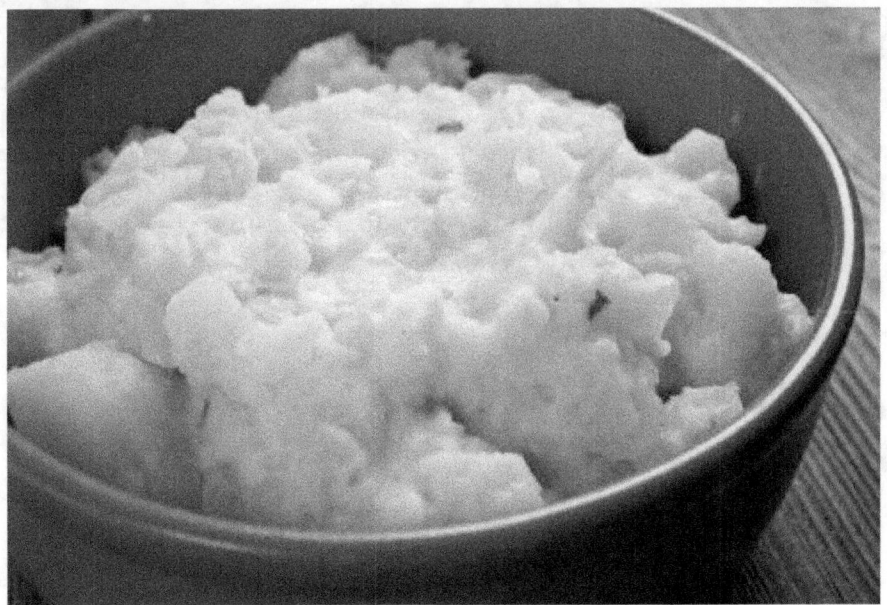

Greece is also very rich in vegetables, including artichokes, cabbages, eggplants, celery, and roots. You can also get plenty of green beans, marrows, potatoes and beans and pulses here. The traditional cuisine normally uses vine leaves as a wrapping for savory meats.

Some of this country's vegetables were brought to her by the conquering warriors of her own cities and states, just as some of the vegetables of southern Spain were brought there by the Moors, who also happened to be extremely accomplished and superb agriculturalists.

The vegetarian bounty of northern Spain is also very well achieved with broad beans, which are usually cooked in oil. Also, dishes made up of aubergine, and tomatoes in a sauce base and spinach and artichokes in different and unusual dish combinations are all mixed up with multicolored vegetables, diced and spiced with wine, chopped ham and Herbs.

And if you do not get access to fresh vegetables, there are always fermented, pickled, preserved, and now frozen vegetables easily available to you.

Why Cook Vegetables in Slices

For a long time, people who did not bother much about using vegetables in fine cuisine just fried them, chopped them or boiled them to death, in oceans of water. There is always a good reason why the Chinese, who are first-rate vegetable cooks vary the angle of their knives and the thickness of the slices when they are cutting up vegetables.

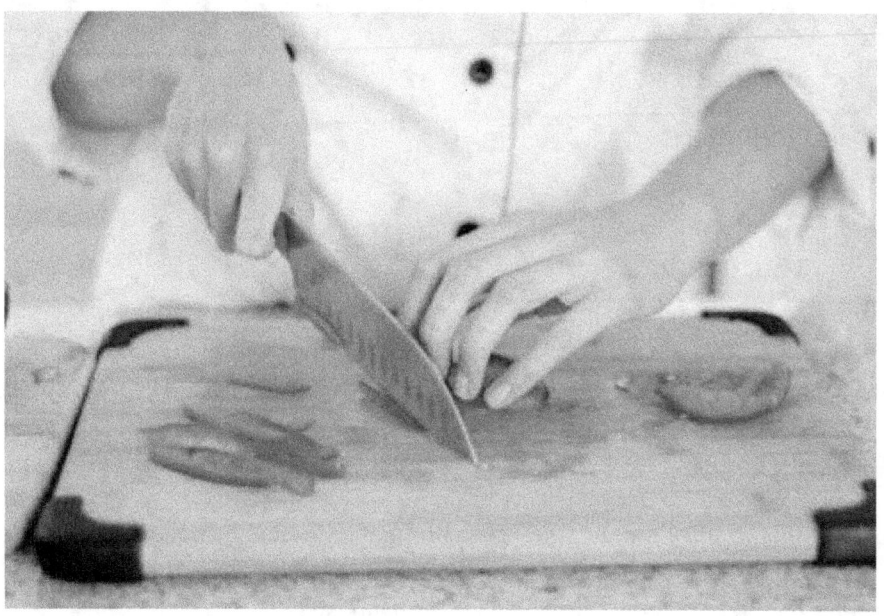

Sometimes their aim is to expose as many surfaces as possible, and sometimes they want to cut with them against the grain of the vegetable to induce nuances of flavor, as well as texture.

Vegetable cookery cannot be done properly without the use of fat and water. So if you have the habit of eating boiled vegetables, you may try braising them instead.

Vegetables and cereal combinations with flavor enhanced by sauces made of herbs and spices have long been eaten traditionally, especially in societies which are based on agricultural communities.

Leaf wrapped Foods

For millenniums, human beings have been using leaves, especially vine leaves. And then those leaves of other greens like spinach, beat, and cabbage which have been used to enfold packets of food. The names for these packets include Dolma[1], Holubtsi, Golabki etc.

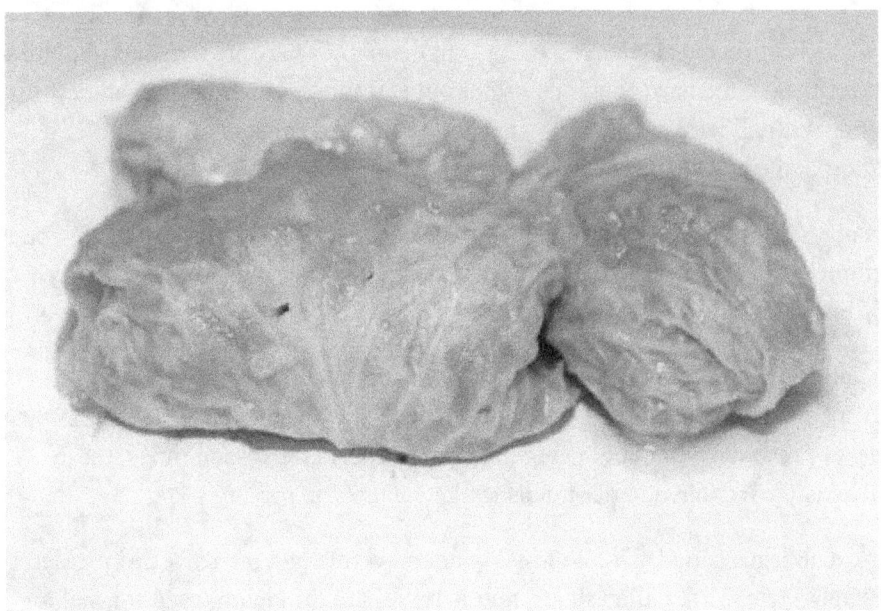

Golabki is a traditional Polish dish.

---

[1] I recall with fondness a really nice French professor of mine named Dolma. Being rather tactless, I could not resist a smile the moment I heard her name. Fortunately, she had a sense of humor, and she told me, "Do not let on what my name means, will you, because everyone thinks it really unique and exotic." And she told me that her father had named her that because she had been such a packet and bundle of mischief, when she was a kid.

One cannot really do anything about the wicked sense of humor of a number of supposedly responsible parents, can one? Well, one can only be glad that he did not name her Holubtsi. In such a case, one would spend a lot of time in her classes, wondering how to pronounce her name, or what it meant! Incidentally, other traditional names for these little packets of food mean "Little pigeon"in the vernacular.

These leaf wrapped foods are generally cooked in meat stock with lemon or tomato juice and served as a side dish. Or they are served as main dishes for lunch and supper.

Fillings and wrappings are going to vary with the seasons, but all of them are cooked for two or three hours to blend in the flavors. These rolls are served either hot or cold.

You can also scalp. The leaves are or boil them until they are soft and pliable. With cabbage, the hard center rib is cut out and the leaves are flattened before filling. With all leaves, roll them around the filling to make a firm bundle, folding in the ends to secure the contents.

It is not necessary to skewer them, but you can also use kitchen string, or wooden toothpicks for fastening, if you feel you must. Trim the ends to make them uniform in size.

It is advisable to line a big dish with large leaves, before the rolls go on to prevent any sort of sticking to the bottom, and to place the leaves on top of the rolls, to prevent drying out during the cooking period. In olden times, these packages were cooked under hot ashes, or steamed in boiling water.

Large cabbages can also be hollowed out and whole and the leaves of pickled cabbage – which are called sauerkraut leaves – are frequently used for making rolls.

Here is the Czechoslovakian way of making cabbage rolls.

Traditional Cabbage Rolls

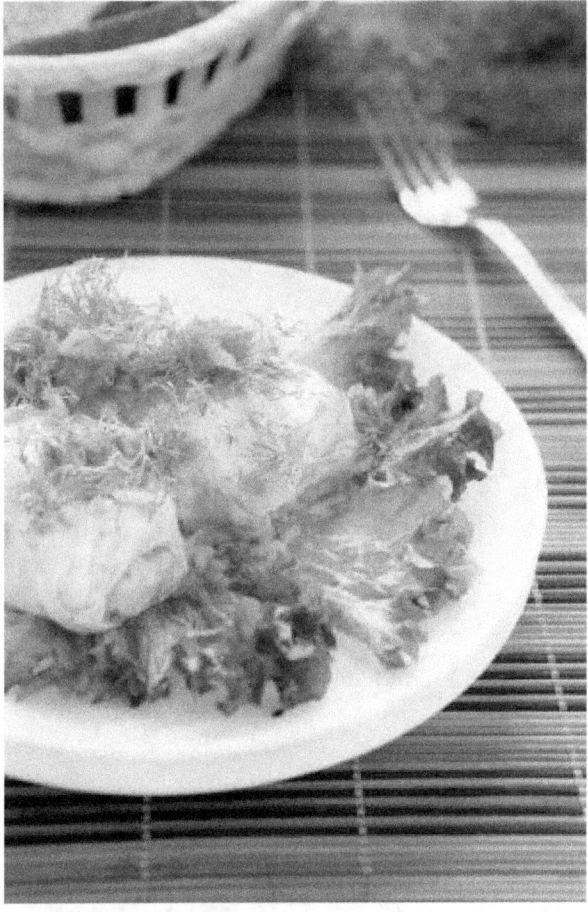

These cabbage leaves, which are stuffed, browned in fat, then cooked in meat or bouillon stock are a popular traditional main meal dish.

For these rolls, you need one fresh cabbage, boiling water, 1 cup raw rice, 2 cups of boiling water – extra –, one teaspoonful of salt, one onion, chopped fine, 2 tablespoons full of bacon fat or dripping, salt and pepper, and extra 3 tablespoons full of bacon fat or dripping, 2 cups bouillon or meat stock and half a cup of sour cream

Remove the core from the cabbage. Cover with boiling water, and leave to stand until the leaves are soft and pliable.

Drain and remove the leaves. Cut out the hard center rib.

Wash the rice, drain, add to boiling water with salt, bring to boil and cook for one minute. Cover tightly, remove from the heat, and let stand until the water is absorbed. This is going to take 15 minutes.

Fry the onion in the bacon fat or the dripping until it is tender. Stir in the rice, season the taste with salt and pepper. Place a heaping teaspoonful of the filling on each leaf and roll tightly. Brown each roll in bacon fat and arranging heavy saucepan.

Mix sour cream, and meat stock, and pour over rolls. Cover and simmer slowly for two hours. Add more stock if necessary.

Sauerkraut

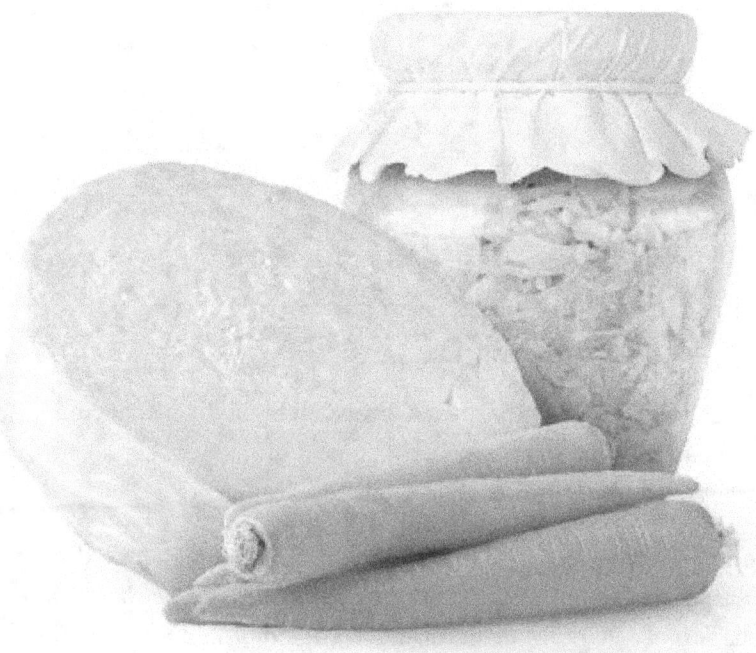

Sauerkraut in Germany, kimchi in Korea – whatever the name, it goes by, this is the traditional way in which you can because cabbage, preserved partly by salting and partly by fermentation. In fact, kimchi is one of the most popular of dishes in Korea, and there is also a museum in Seoul, – Pulmuone kimchi museum, which opened its doors in 1986 – which concentrates only on the different forms of kimchi recipes, which have come down through different regions and down the ages.

Along with sauerkraut, kimchi is also a traditional fermented cabbage dish, which is very popular in Korean cuisine. In fact, there is a museum dedicated to the more than 600 traditional kimchi recipes and preparations in Seoul.

Nevertheless, the basic ingredients are always going to be cabbage and salt, whether you are making sauerkraut or you are making kimchi.

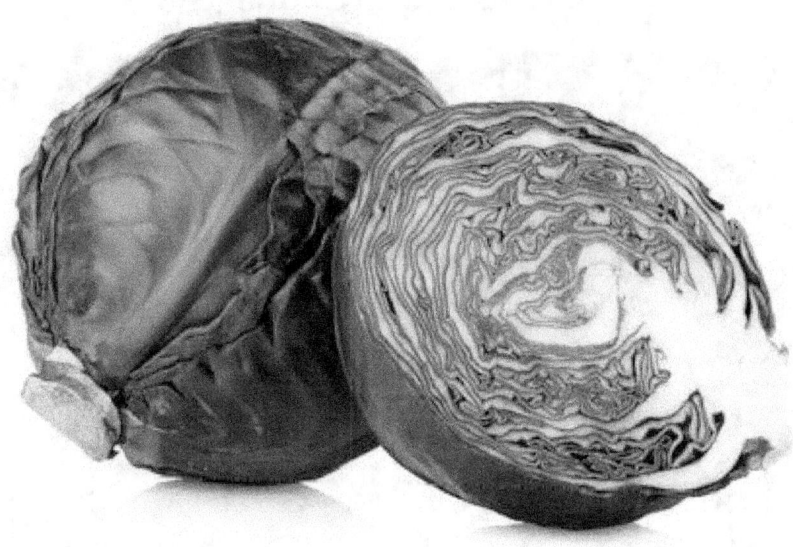

Kimchi can be made up of red cabbage, but white cabbage has been used on the ages.

You may want to use the hard and white cabbage for making sauerkraut.

Trim the cabbage, cut into four, removed most of the hard stalks, then cut down into thin and fine shreds.

Pack into a large wooden tub or stone crock in layers with salt in proportion of not more than about two – 3 ounces per 5 pounds of cabbage.

Cover the top with cabbage leaves, press down well.

Cover with a piece of muslin and put a wooden board on the top with a heavy weight on it. Leave in a warm place – between 17 and 78°F [21 and 25°C] for 2 to 3 weeks to allow fermentation to take place.

Drain off the liquid. If the sauerkraut is not for immediate use, back into boxing charts when all the fermentation has seized and sterilize for 40 minutes with the lid on the pan and the bottles were screwed or. Keep in a cool place until required.

Kimchi-or Fermented Radish/Cabbage

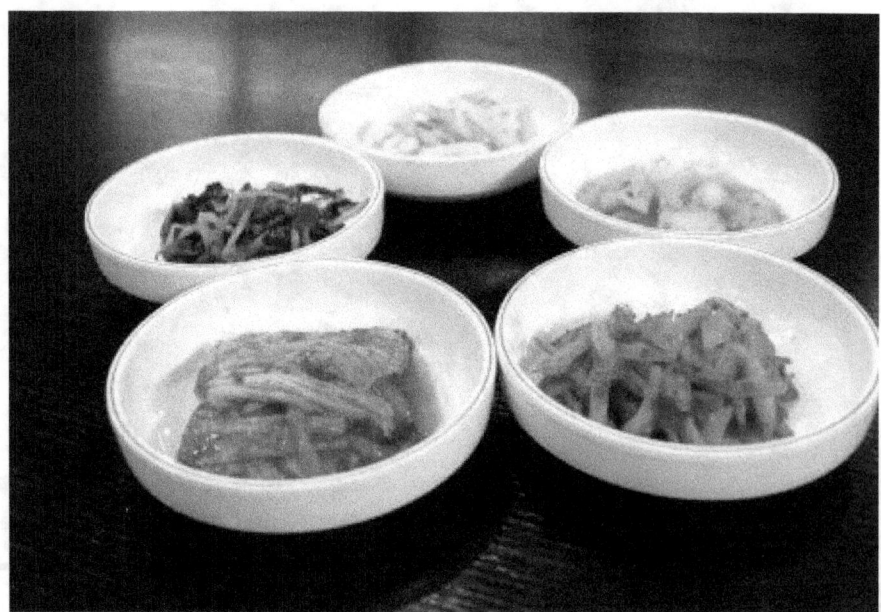

Traditional Korean Kimchi Made Up Of Different Vegetables

Kimchi is getting to be known as one of the most popular of traditional and ancient Korean dishes, in the West. Thanks to its healthy ingredients, subtle flavorings, sour, sweet and spicy taste, the national dish of Korea is now being presented here, for your good health.

Early Kimchi was made up of cabbage and meat stock in ancient times. Red peppers were not introduced until the 14 century by the Japanese, and soon, they became an integral part of the Kimchi, to give it a hot flavor. There is a museum in Seoul dedicated totally to kimchi, which has 187 current as well as historic varieties versions and recipes of this dish.

The ingredients are one Chinese cabbage, but you can also use four radishes or turnips. This is going to be mixed Kimchi.
One small clove of garlic, as well as a tiny piece of chopped ginger, – the same quantity as the garlic.
One Apple -cooking
4 tablespoons full of red chili powder – it is going to be hot!
2 tablespoons full of sugar
Chop the Chinese cabbage, radish and turnips, into small squares.
When you have finished chopping up all the vegetables, place all of these pieces in a glass pickle container. Add salt, so that all the liquid can get absorbed but do not add so much of the salt so that this recipe becomes thoroughly inedible.

You may want to use your own estimate. Consider yourself making pickles.

Cover the container with its air tight lid. Place in the sun in a shady place. Kimchi is ready within one day, in summer, but it needs three days of winter sun, depending on the level of the humidity and the temperature.

The radish and the cabbage is going to dry out within a couple of days, thanks to the salt. Now grate the Apple, garlic and ginger and place it in a container.

The ingredients, which are going to be using now are the garlic, ginger, Apple, red chili powder, salt and sugar.

Boil a glass of water, and pour it in the bowl, in which you have put the salt, red chili powder and the sugar. This water is excellent for mixing all these items. Now add the grated mixture to this sugar, chili powder mixture.

Add the sun dried and salted cabbage/radish a little by little.to this liquid, stirring all the while. This kimchi can be eaten now, but I would suggest allowing it to ferment a little more for some days. It is going to be even tastier.

Kimchi is delicious eaten fresh or eaten preserved. Kimchi is normally served with rice and meat. Try this way of eating kimchi. Take a little bit of meat, top it up with hot kimchi, pop it in your mouth, and cool yourself down with a mouth full of bland rice. Do not eat it by itself. You can also try kimchi sandwiches, by layering some bread with meat, kimchi, green lettuce, butter, cheese, tomatoes and cucumber. Talk about subs!

Also, try kimchi omelette, where you are going to eat eggs with chopped onions, spices and seasonings, and made piquant with kimchi.

Artichokes

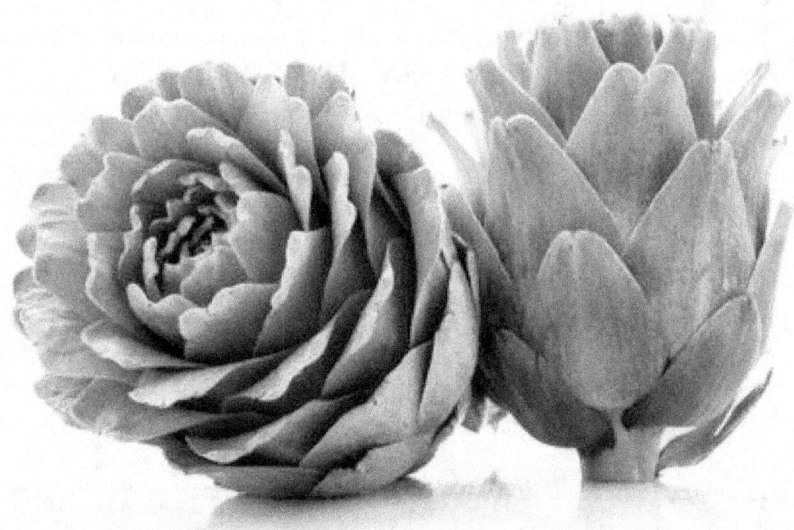

There was once upon a time when artichoke was considered to be the most expensive of all garden products. However, in medieval times, artichokes were commonly grown in all well-stocked, Elizabethan gardens in England. Luckily now, fresh artichokes, appearing quite frequently in your market are not too expensive. And the best thing about them is that they are going to become a delicacy, just with a simple sauce.

There are number of ways of preparing artichokes. You can stuff them with meat or vegetables, and bake or steam them. You can dip the hearts in fritter batter and fry them up in hot fat. You can serve them cold, indifferent, salads.

In Haute cuisine, the heart of an artichoke is considered to be an indispensable garnish.

Choosing and Eating Artichokes

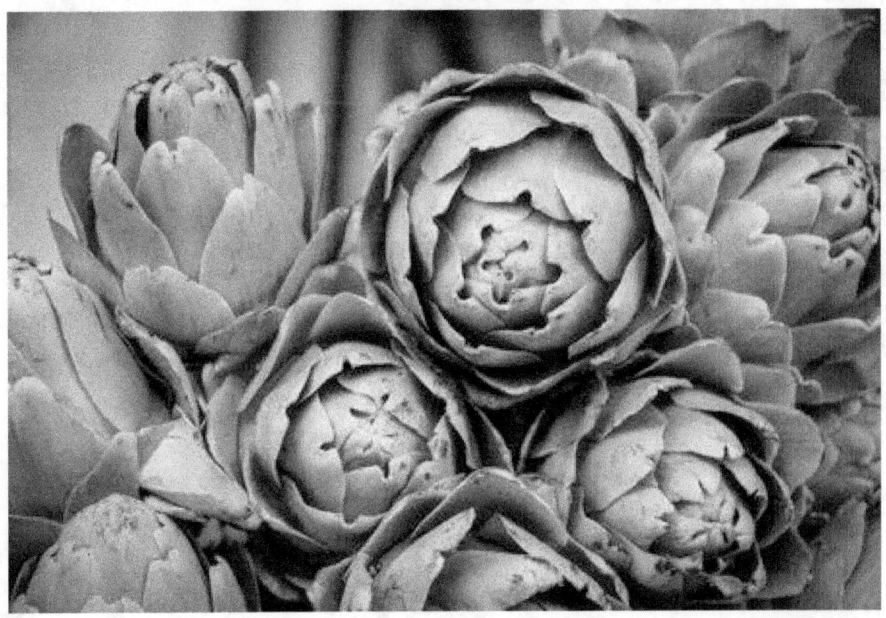

If you are eating artichokes for the first time, you need to choose compact and heavy globes. They should be fresh, dark green, with tightly clinging scales. You can allow one large artichoke for each person, or two smaller ones.

Wash in several changes of water, to get rid of all the dust and possible pesticides, and cut off about half an inch of the leaves with scissors. Also, the vigorous scrubbing is needed because the many protuberances in the artichoke globe is going to make peeling difficult.

Tie the artichokes with thread to secure the leaves and cook in boiling water with a tablespoonful of salt and the juice of one lemon for one hour or until they are tender. Remove the strings and place upside down to drain.

Serve hot with the melted butter seasoned with pepper.

The artichoke is eaten by pulling off each leaf and dipping it in white sauce. Only the stalk end of the leaf is eaten. The rest is discarded.

When the leaves have all been removed, the hairy growth, which is known as the choke is cut off to reveal the heart, which is the choicest spot. This is eaten with a fork.

White Sauce for Artichokes

For this White sauce, you need 3 tablespoons full of butter, one tablespoonful of flour, 1 cup of water, salted water, salt and pepper to taste, 2 egg yolks and juice of one lemon.

Melt the butter, blend in the flour, add the water gradually and cook until all the liquid has thickened. Add the pepper and salt to taste.

Remove from heat and stir in the yolks of two eggs, beaten up with lemon juice. Strain and pour over the artichokes. Or you can dip the leaves in this sauce and eat.

Peas

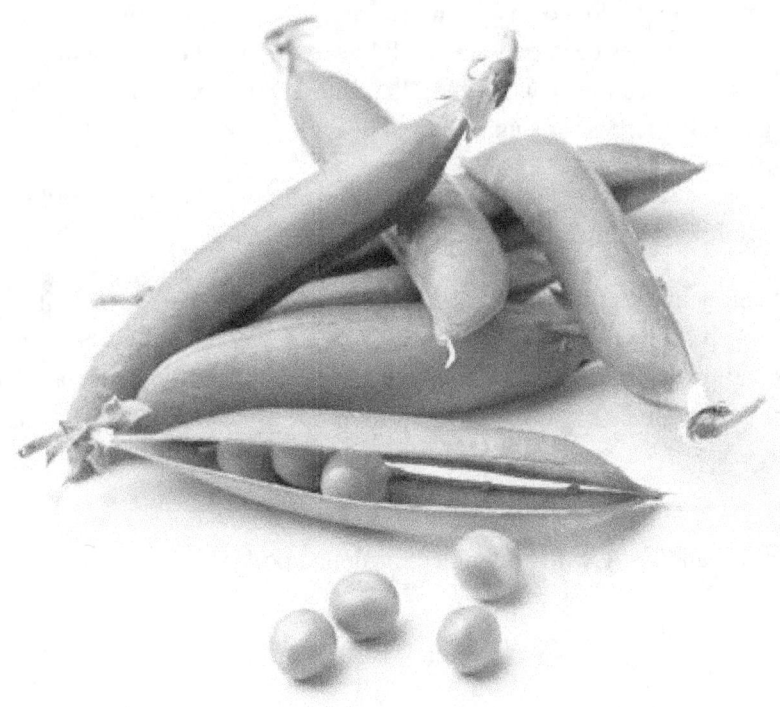

We are lucky to find these delicious vegetables, easily and all over the world. They appear in company with lettuce in a cream sauce in Hungary and Austria. When fresh peas are not available, you are going to get them in the shape of peas pudding. In many parts of Europe, green peas are cooked with garlic, onion, nutmeg, and Bay. They can also be flavored with cloves, sugar and vinegar before garnishing with a sprinkling of parsley, and then served.

All kinds of European vegetable puddings, either steamed or baked blend the chosen vegetables in layers with layers of egg or other ingredients like herbs, potatoes, and even chopped meat.

Traditional Peas Pudding

This dish is normally served with boiled beef and boiled pork in England. British cuisine has been overlooked by the more enterprising and adventurous French cooks, down the ages because the British have a habit of boiling all the vegetables on which they can lay their hands. So naturally, traditional peas pudding is going to be made up of boiled peas.

For this you need 3 cups of split peas, cold water, 4 tablespoons full of butter, and pepper and salt to taste.

Soak the peas in the cold water overnight. Drain, and tie them loosely in a cloth, leaving room for them to swell up. Place in a deep pan of cold water, bring to a boil, and allow to cook for 3 hours. Drain and rub through colander, add butter, salt and pepper, and beat well. Tie it tightly in the cloth which has been lightly floured

Place in a pan of boiling water, and allow to boil for one hour. Turn out on serving dish and serve with boiled beef or boiled pork.[2]

---

[2] *There, the boiling procedure again, even for meat. Well, each to his own.*

Dolma

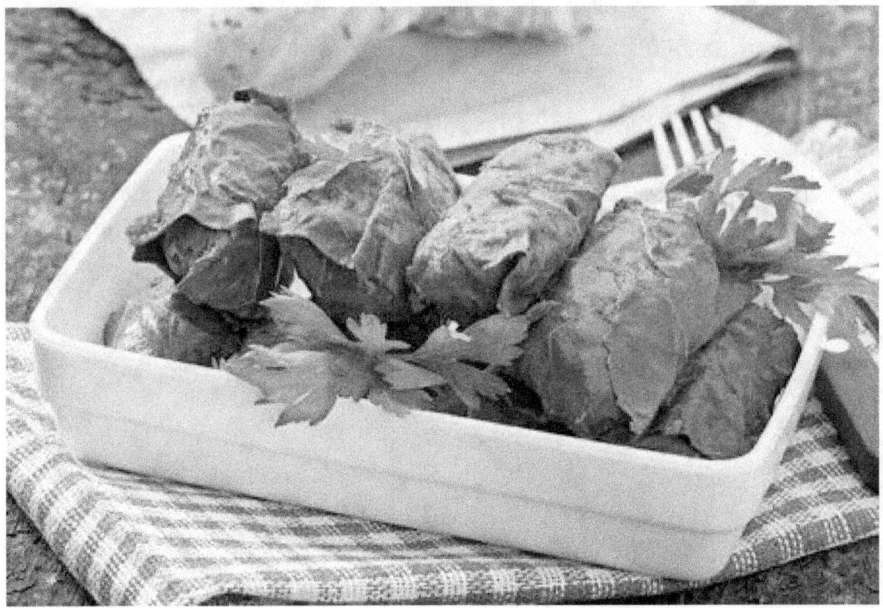

This is originally a Greek dish, which is made up of Rice, seasoned with mint and thyme, and other herbs, and then wrapped in vine leaves. If you do not get them fresh, you can purchase these leaves in tins. Serve cold with wedges of lemon.

For these packages, you need half a cup of olive oil, two onions, finely chopped, 1 cup of rice, 1 ½ cups of hot water, ¼ cup of pine nuts or kernels, ¼ cups of currants, one teaspoonful of chopped mint, half a teaspoonful of thyme, one teaspoonful of sugar, salt and pepper to taste, 3 tablespoons full of tomato purée, one tablespoonful of olive oil, hot water, juice of one lemon, and 40 fresh grape leaves. Or 1 tin of vine leaves.

Sauté the onions in the olive oil over medium heat until tender. Add the rice and sauté until it turns yellow. This is going to take about 15 minutes. Keep stirring constantly. Put in the water, pine kernels, currants, mint, thyme, sugar, salt, pepper and tomato purée.

Cover and simmer for about 20 minutes, until the liquid is absorbed and the rice is tender. Cool.

Pour the boiling water over the vine leaves, leave to stand for a few minutes until pliable. If you are using the leaves from a tin, just wash them, and then drain.

Place a teaspoonful of stuffing on each leaf, roll up neatly and arrange in layers or in well-greased fireproof pans. Sprinkle with lemon juice and olive oil, and pour in enough of hot water to cover the dolmas.

Put an inverted plate over them, to keep them in place. Cover tightly and simmer over low heat for two hours. Remove from heat and cool. Serve cold with lemon wedges.

Sauté Fennel

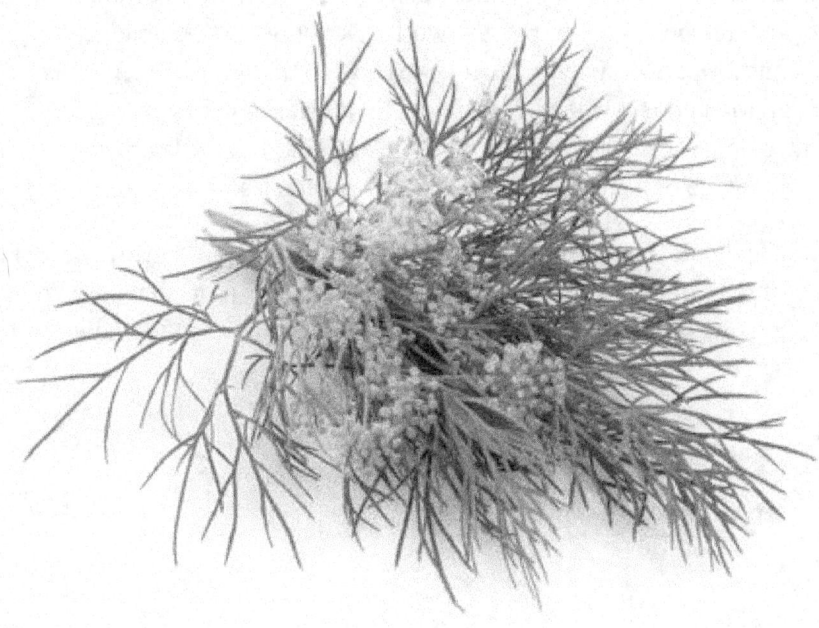

Now this is an unusual dish especially when you use fennel, also known as Anise as an Herb. This has a mild licorice like flavor, and you can eat it raw with been your and oil dressing. You can cook it as a side dish also as it is done in Italy.

For this you need one and a half pounds of fennel. Choose fennel with white hearts and dark green leaves. Wash thoroughly under cold water and remove the tough outer leaves.

You also need 6 cups of water, 1 teaspoon of salt, one crushed garlic, 2 tablespoons full of olive oil and pepper to taste.

Cut the tender fennel leaves in half, and cut the hearts in quarters.

Bring the salt and water to boil, add the fennel, cover and slowly until it is sender. This is going to take 10 minutes. Sauté the garlic in hot oil until it is browned, then remove the garlic from pan and add the fennel.

Sauté for three minutes, dust with pepper, and serve immediately.

Conclusion

This book has just given you a limited look into the world of vegetables with easy to cook recipes from all over the world. Not only are these recipes very healthy, but they also happen to be time-tested and traditional. Man is basically a hunter and forager. But when he found out that it was easier to grow vegetables, he decided on an agricultural society, where he could just settle down in one area, near some source of water, and grow his own vegetables.

Besides, he did not have to stay out every day, with his bow and arrow, looking for elusive fare for the cook pot, when all he had to do was to step out into his garden, and pluck fresh vegetables. So add more vegetables to your diet, and live a healthier life.

Live Long and Prosper!

Author Bio

Dueep Jyot Singh is a Management and IT Professional who managed to gather Postgraduate qualifications in Management and English and Degrees in Science, French and Education while pursuing different enjoyable career options like being an hospital administrator, IT,SEO and HRD Database Manager/ trainer, movie , radio and TV scriptwriter, theatre artiste and public speaker, lecturer in French, Marketing and Advertising, ex-Editor of Hearts On Fire (now known as Solstice) Books Missouri USA, advice columnist and cartoonist, publisher and Aviation School trainer, ex- moderator on Medico.in, banker, student councilor ,travelogue writer … among other things!

One fine morning, she decided that she had enough of killing herself by Degrees and went back to her first love -- writing. It's more enjoyable! She already has 48 published academic and 14 fiction- in- different- genre books under her belt.

When she is not designing websites or making Graphic design illustrations for clients , she is browsing through old bookshops hunting for treasures, of which she has an enviable collection – including R.L. Stevenson, O.Henry, Dornford Yates, Maurice Walsh, De Maupassant, Victor Hugo, Sapper, C.N. Williamson, "Bartimeus" and the crown of her collection- Dickens "The Old Curiosity Shop," and so on… Just call her "Renaissance Woman") - collecting herbal remedies, acting like Universal Helping Hand/Agony Aunt, or escaping to her dear mountains for a bit of exploring, collecting herbs and plants and trekking.

1. Amazon.com
2. Barnes and Noble
3. Itunes
4. Kobo
5. Smashwords
6. Google Play Books

Check out some of the other JD-Biz Publishing books

Gardening Series on Amazon

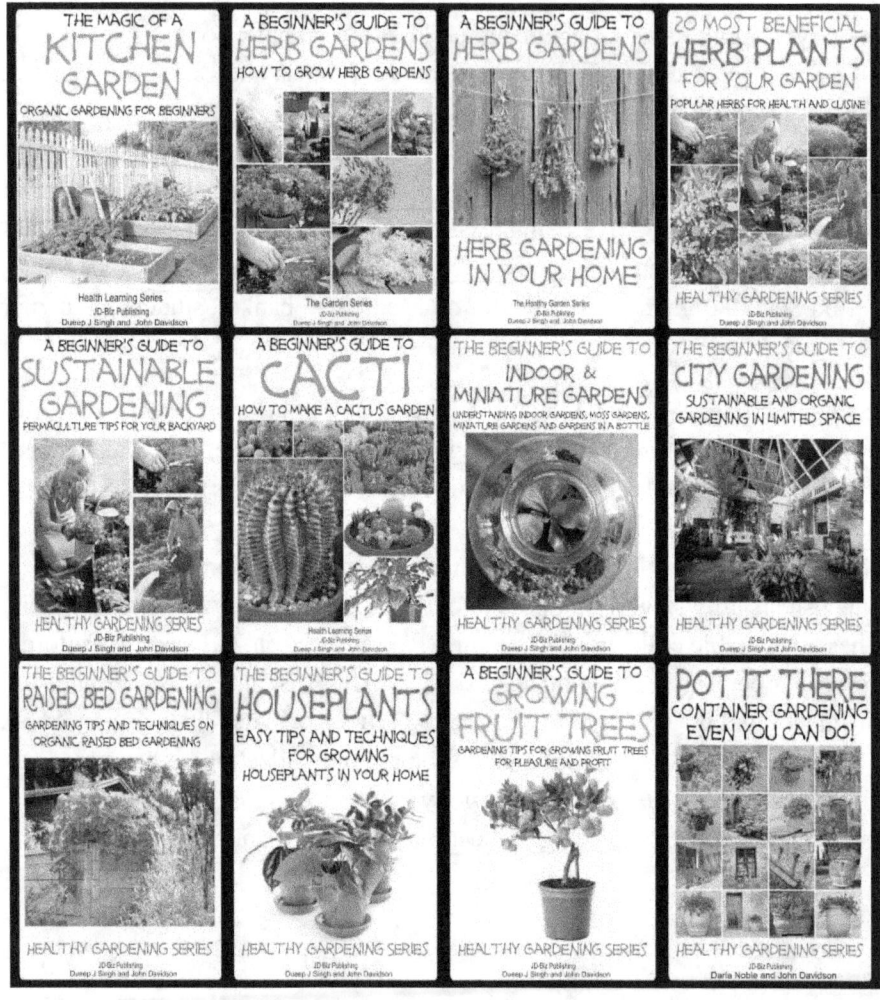

THE MAGIC OF GOOSEBERRIES FOR HEALTH AND BEAUTY | THE MAGIC OF YOGURT FOR COOKING AND BEAUTY | THE MAGIC OF LEMONS USING LEMONS FOR HEALTH AND BEAUTY | THE MAGIC OF CHILLIES FOR COOKING AND HEALING | THE MAGIC OF ONIONS ONIONS IN CUISINE TO CURE AND TO HEAL | THE MAGIC OF RADISHES TO CURE AND TO HEAL

THE MAGIC OF CARROTS TO CURE AND TO HEAL | THE HEALTH BENEFITS OF OREGANO FOR COOKING AND HEALTH | THE MAGIC OF MARIGOLDS Marigolds for Health And Beauty | THE HEALTH BENEFITS OF CINNAMON FOR COOKING AND HEALING | THE MAGIC OF COCONUTS FOR COOKING & HEALTH | THE MAGIC OF CLOVES FOR HEALING AND COOKING

THE MAGIC OF ASAFETIDA FOR COOKING AND HEALING | THE MAGIC OF NEEM MARGOSA TO HEAL | THE MAGIC OF SALT TO HEAL AND FOR BEAUTY | THE MAGIC OF POMEGRANATES FOR HEALTH AND BEAUTY | THE MAGIC OF DRY FRUIT AND SPICES REMEDIES AND RECIPES | THE HEALTH BENEFITS OF TURMERIC CURCUMIN FOR COOKING AND HEALTH

THE MAGIC OF ALOE VERA | THE MAGIC OF VEGETABLES ANCIENT HEALING REMEDIES AND TIPS | THE HEALTH BENEFITS OF ROSEMARY FOR COOKING AND HEALTH | THE MAGIC OF PEPPER & PEPPERCORNS FOR COOKING & HEALING | THE MAGIC OF MILK, BUTTER AND CHEESE FOR COOKING & HEALING | THE MAGIC OF CARDAMOMS FOR COOKING AND HEALTH

THE HEALTH BENEFITS OF BLACK CUMIN FOR COOKING AND HEALTH | THE MAGIC OF BASIL-TULSI TO HEAL NATURALLY | THE MAGIC OF SPICES FOR HEALTH AND CUISINE | THE MAGIC OF ROSES FOR COOKING AND BEAUTY | The Miraculous Healing Powers of GINGER | The Miracle of HONEY

Country Life Books

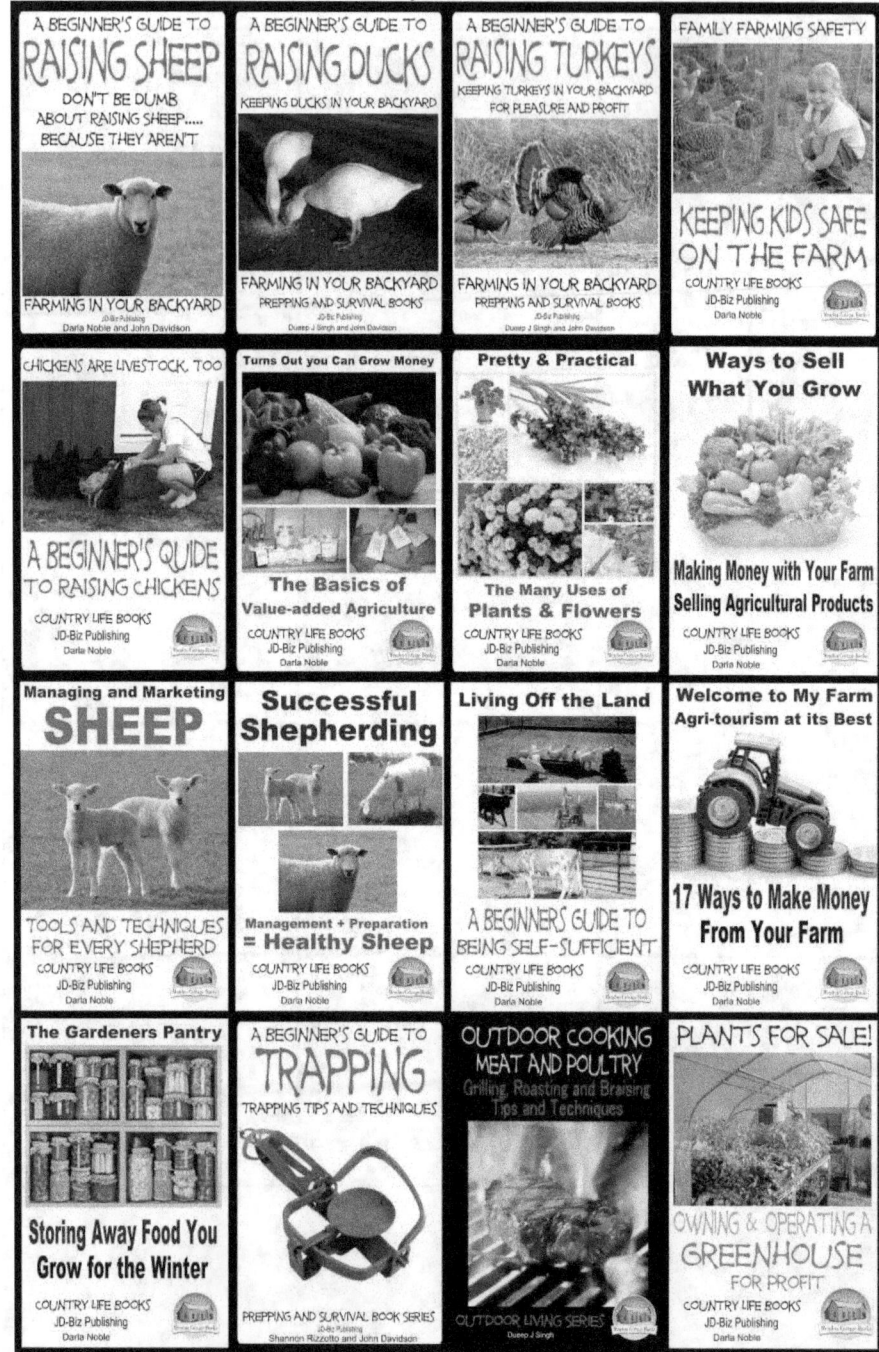

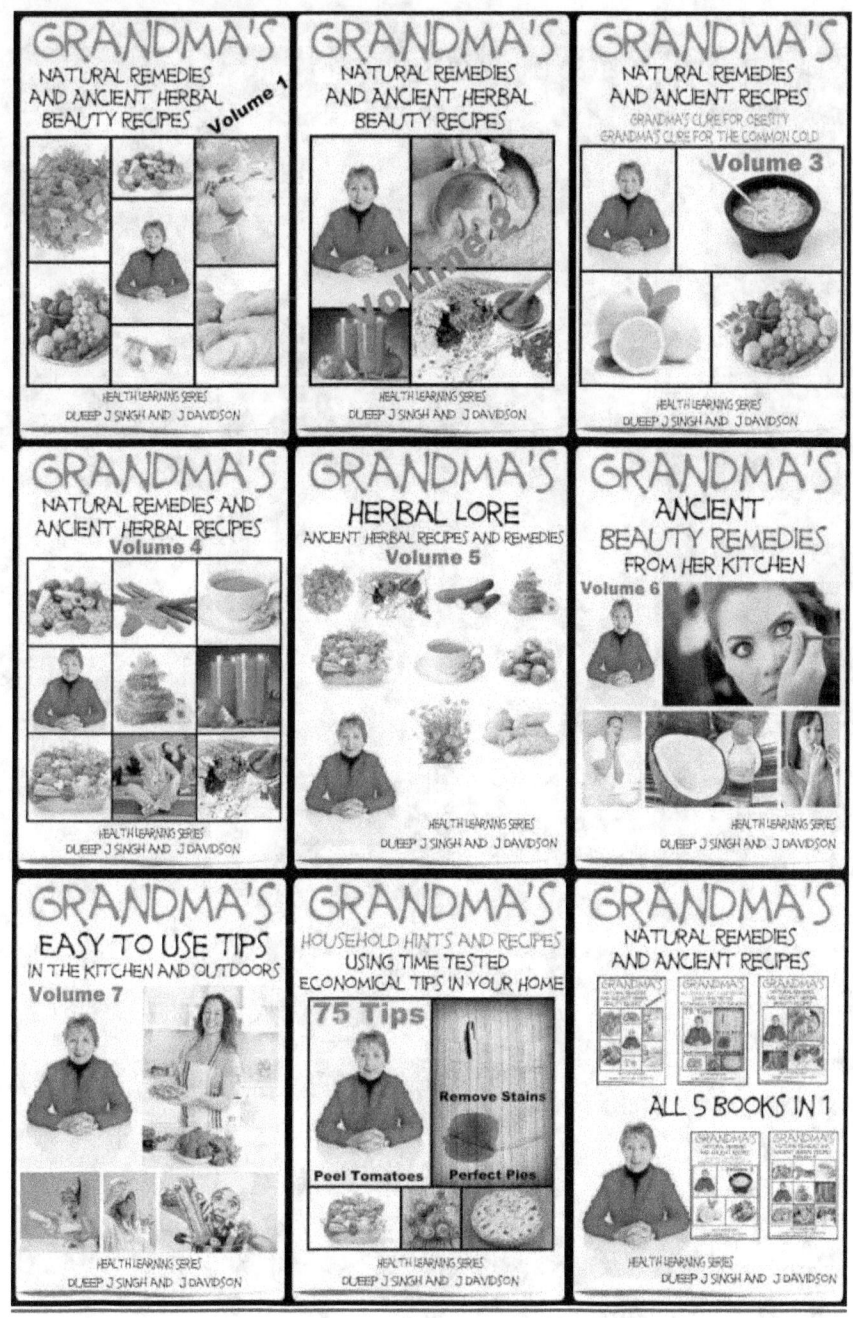

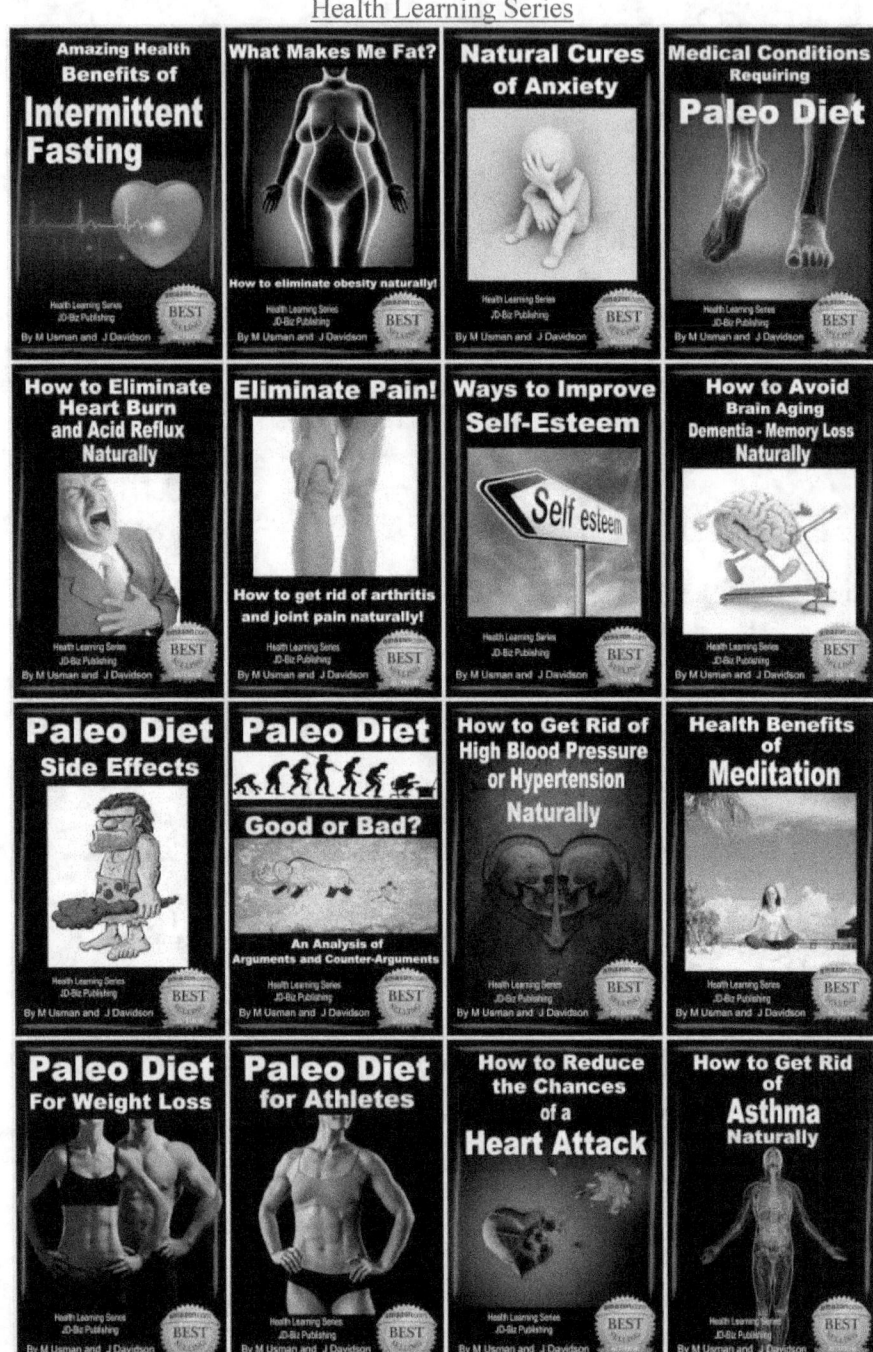

Amazing Animal Book Series

Learn To Draw Series

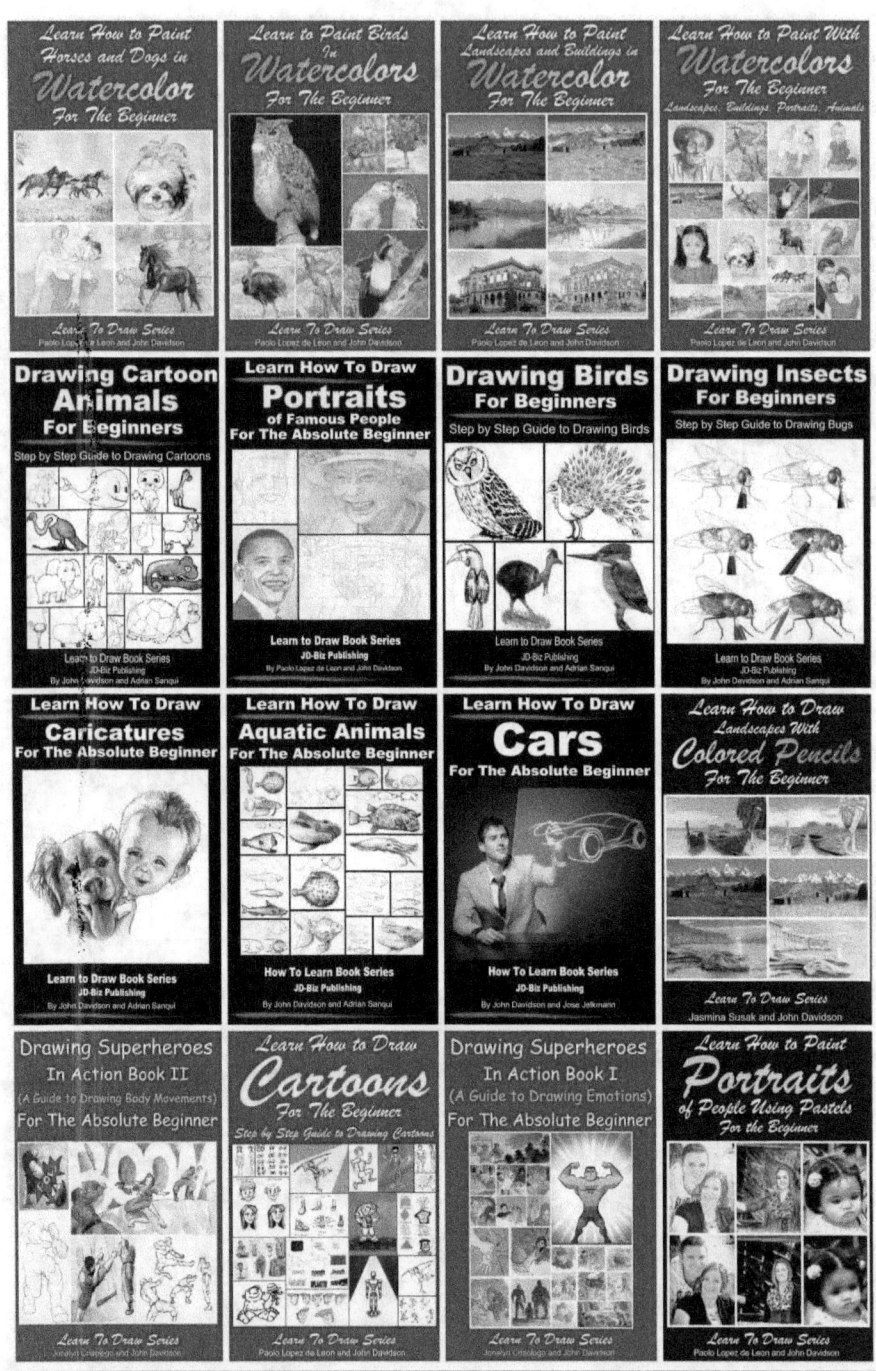

How to Build and Plan Books

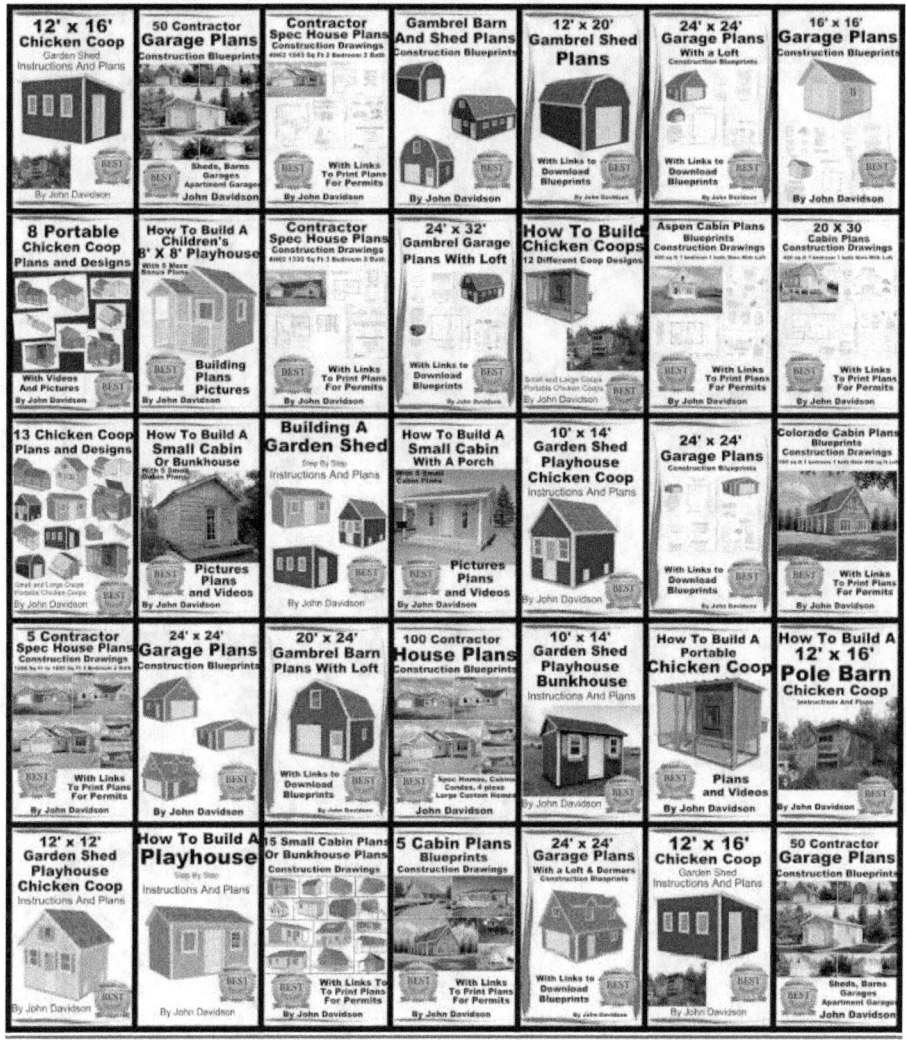

Entrepreneur Book Series

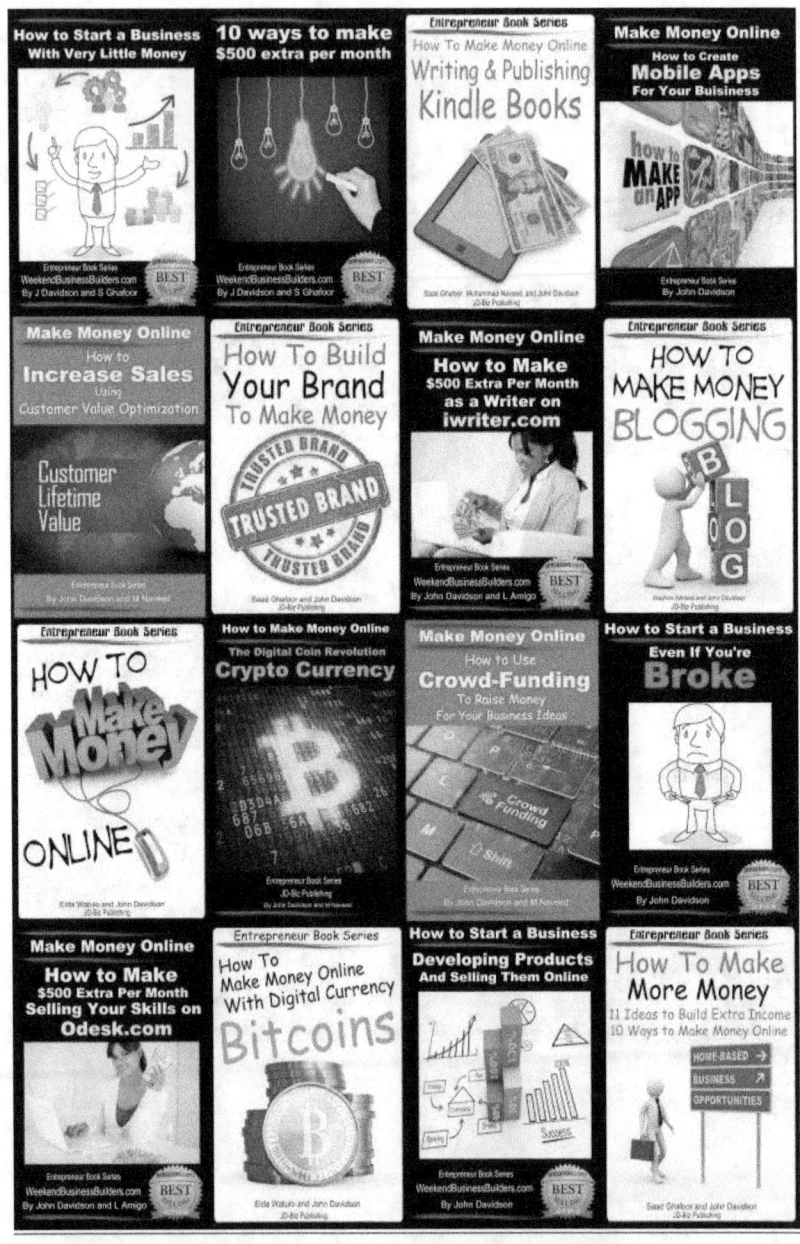

Publisher

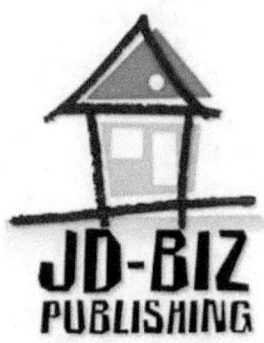

JD-Biz Corp

P O Box 374

Mendon, Utah 84325

http://www.jd-biz.com/

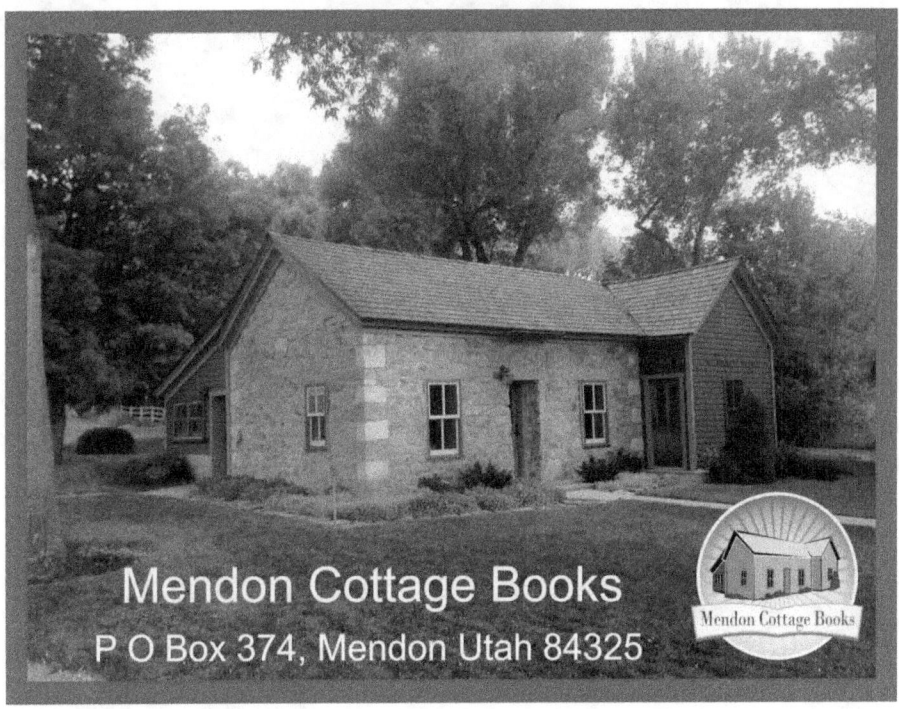

Mendon Cottage Books

P O Box 374, Mendon Utah 84325

www.ingramcontent.com/pod-product-compliance
Lightning Source LLC
Chambersburg PA
CBHW061803280526
45787CB00003BA/1459